DAVID HAS AIDS

The Story by DORIS SANFORD
Illustrations by GRACI EVANS

MULTNOMAH
Portland, Oregon 97266

D1601903

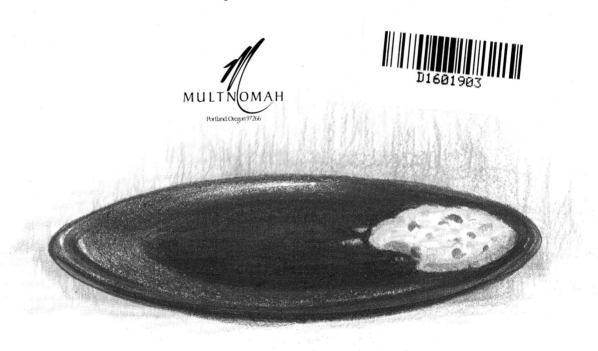

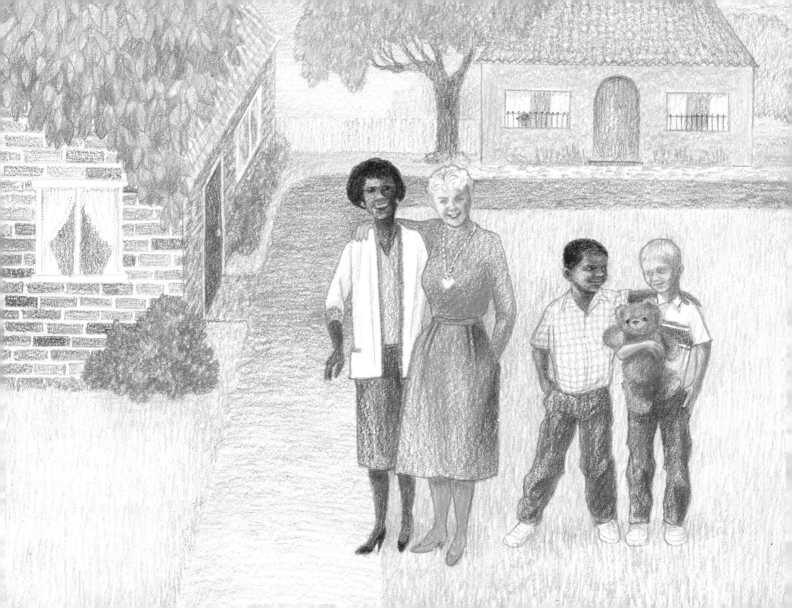

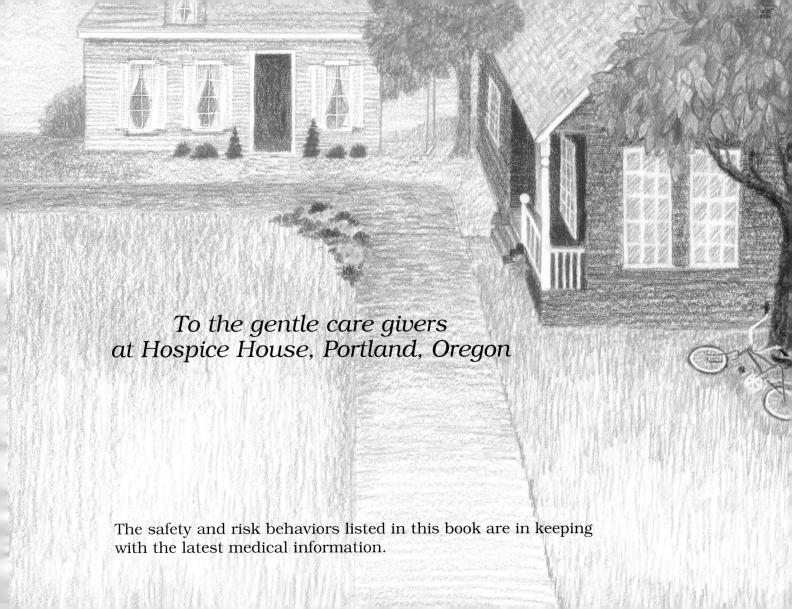

To the gentle care givers
at Hospice House, Portland, Oregon

The safety and risk behaviors listed in this book are in keeping
with the latest medical information.

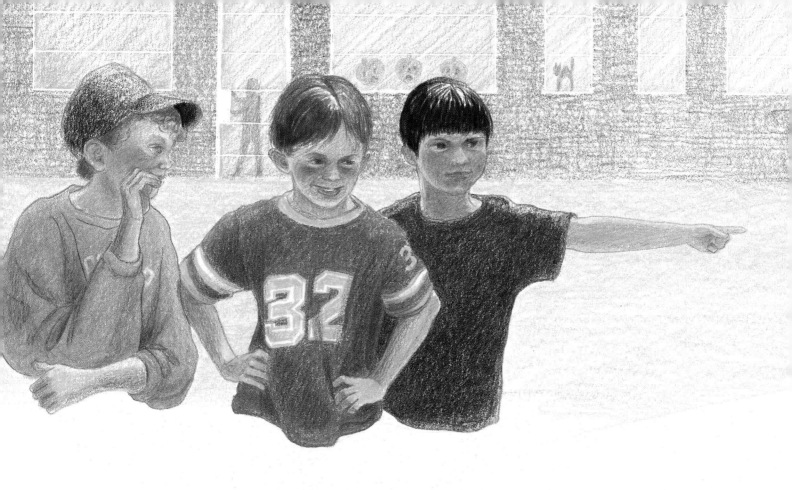

I wish I had a friend . . . somebody to play with me.

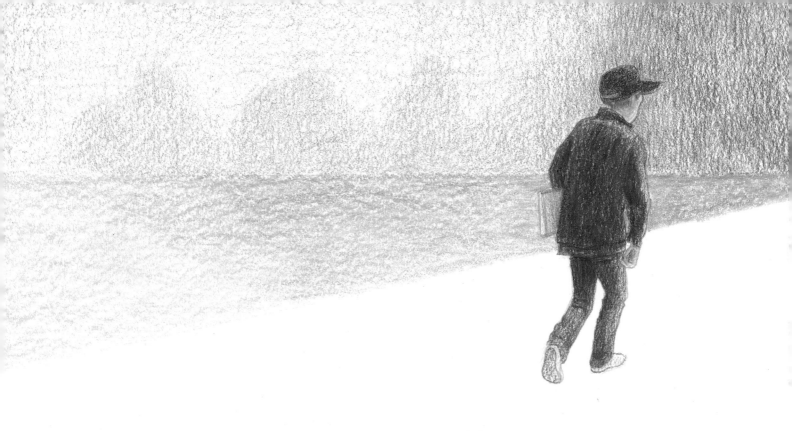

I'm the one in danger, not them! My body is filled with
AIDS, but theirs are filled with fear.

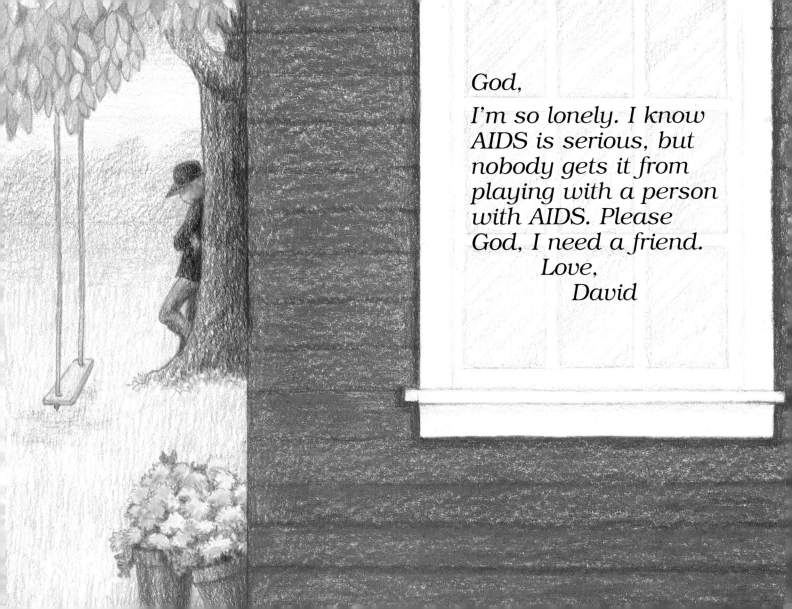

God,

I'm so lonely. I know AIDS is serious, but nobody gets it from playing with a person with AIDS. Please God, I need a friend.
Love,
David

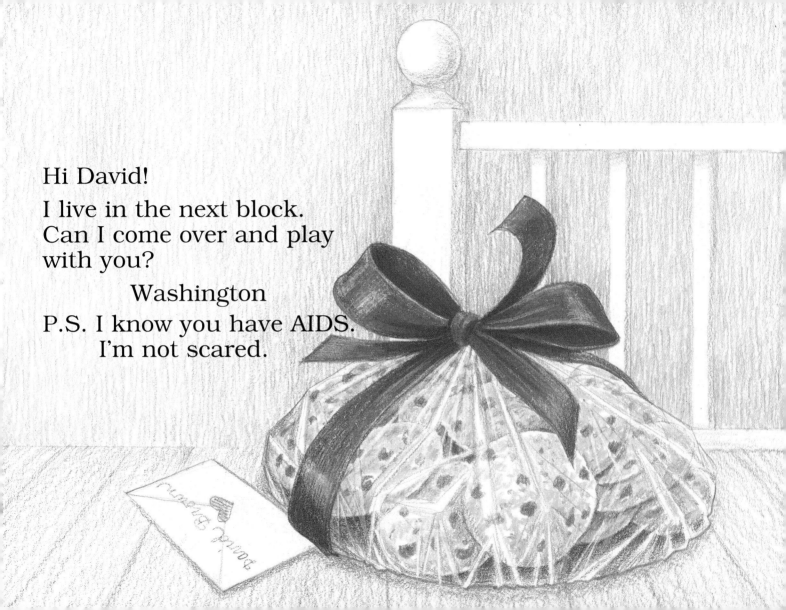

Hi David!

I live in the next block.
Can I come over and play
with you?

       Washington

P.S. I know you have AIDS.
    I'm not scared.

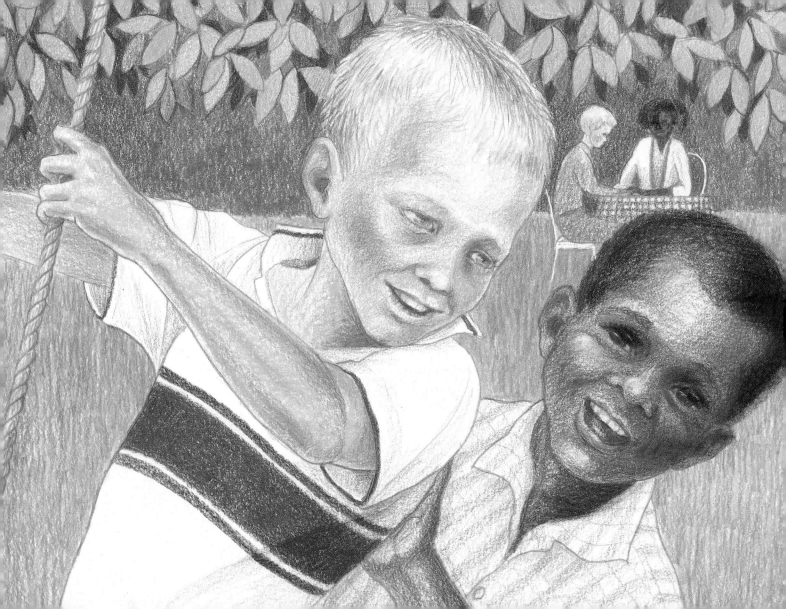

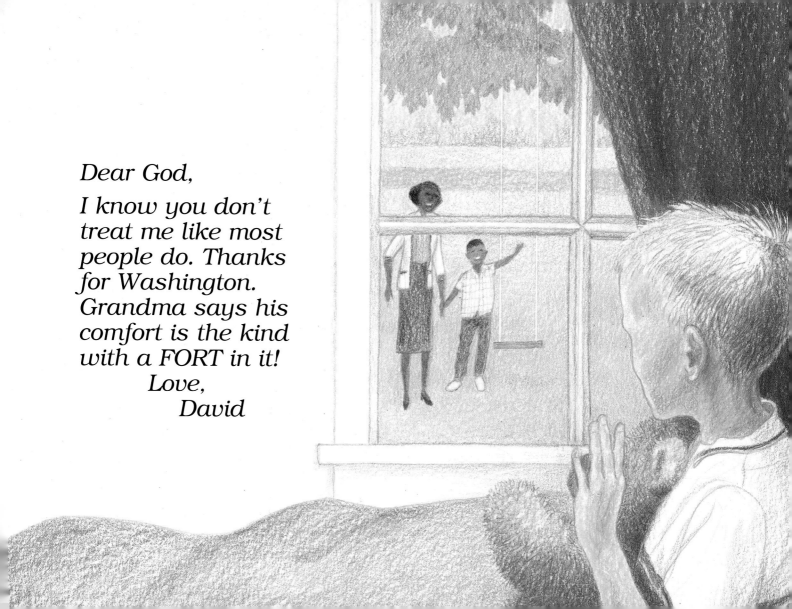

Dear God,

I know you don't treat me like most people do. Thanks for Washington. Grandma says his comfort is the kind with a FORT in it!
Love,
David

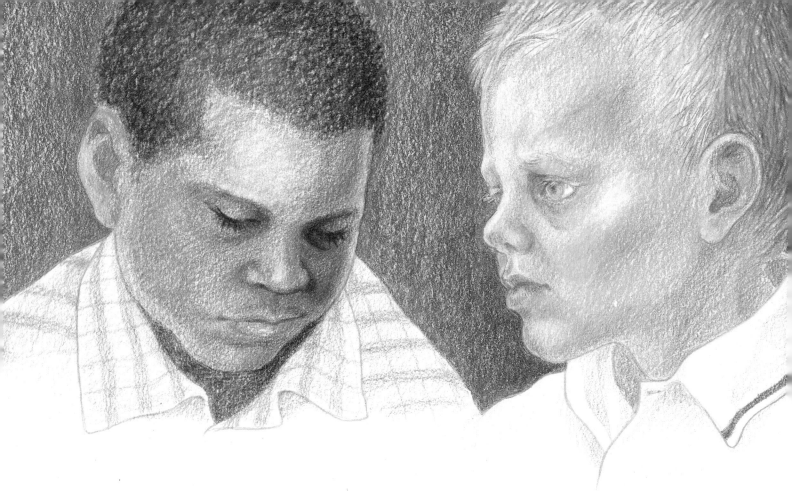

"Why do people worry about me going to school with the other kids? I know the health safety rules for AIDS."

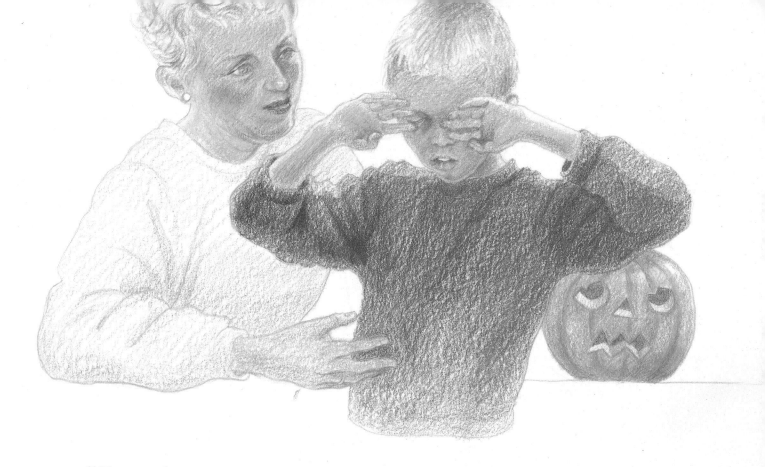

"Grandma, I hate it when I miss special days at
school because I'm sick!"

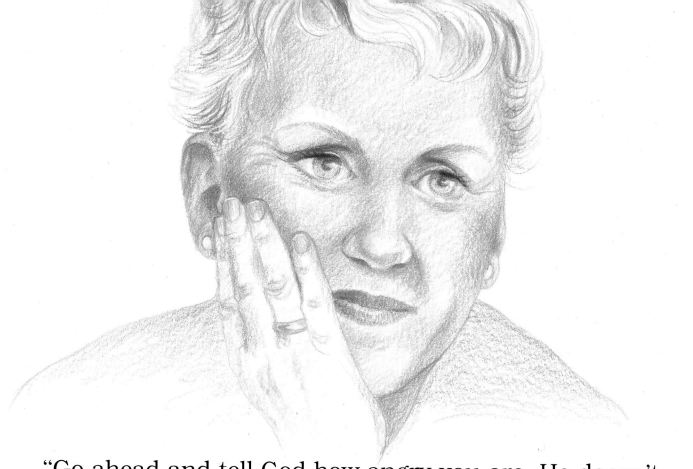

"Go ahead and tell God how angry you are. He doesn't ask you not to feel hurt, angry, or lonely, but to let Him help you no matter *how* you feel."

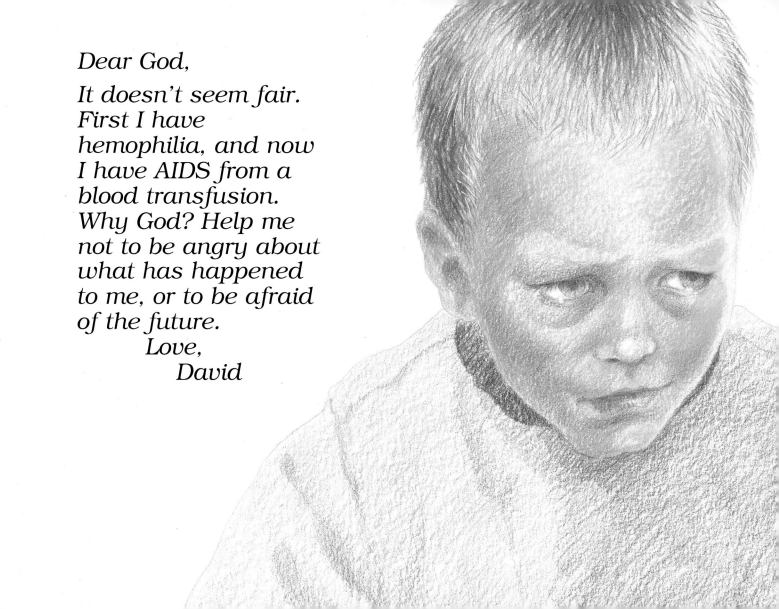

Dear God,

It doesn't seem fair.
First I have
hemophilia, and now
I have AIDS from a
blood transfusion.
Why God? Help me
not to be angry about
what has happened
to me, or to be afraid
of the future.
          Love,
              David

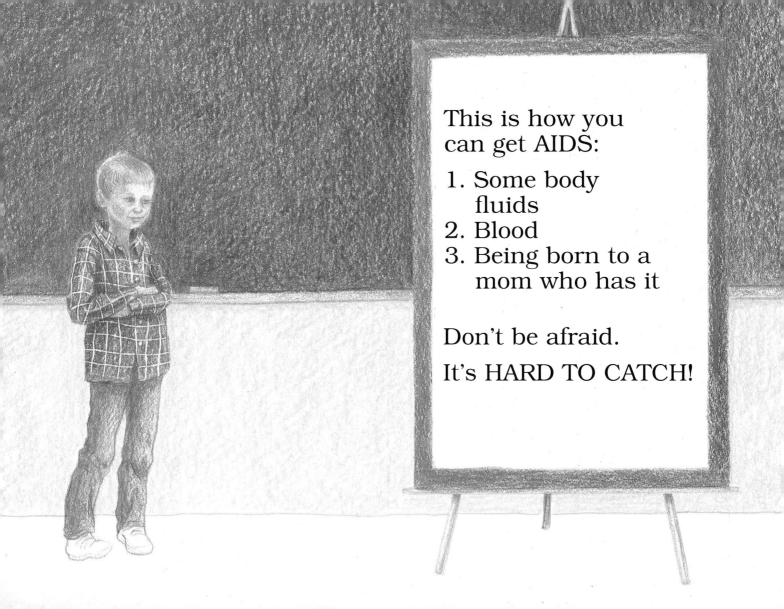

This is how you can get AIDS:

1. Some body fluids
2. Blood
3. Being born to a mom who has it

Don't be afraid.

It's HARD TO CATCH!

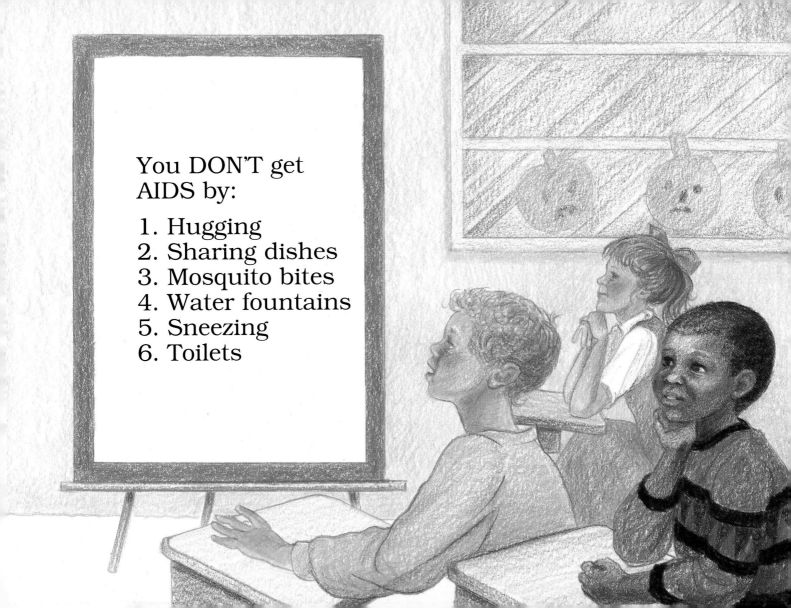

You DON'T get AIDS by:

1. Hugging
2. Sharing dishes
3. Mosquito bites
4. Water fountains
5. Sneezing
6. Toilets

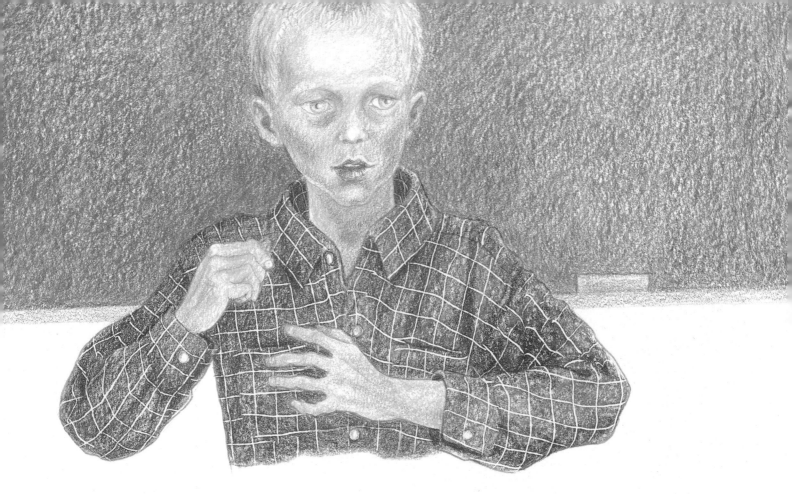

The most dangerous person with AIDS is the one you DON'T know has the disease.

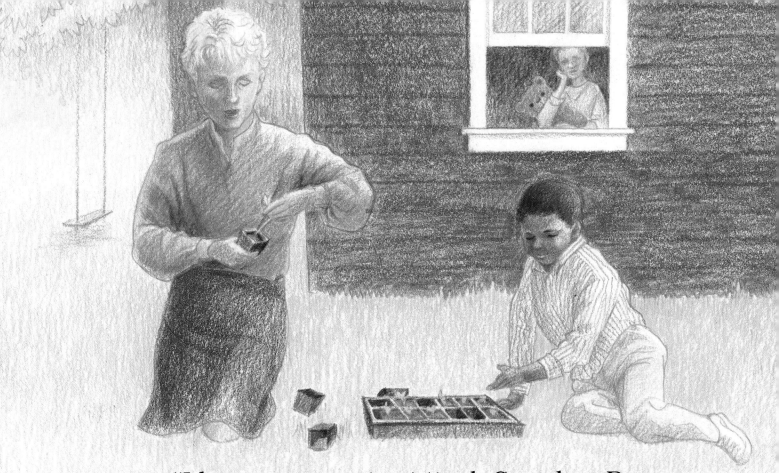

"I know you must get tired, Grandma Brown.
Mom said that one way to help David is to make
it easier for *you*."

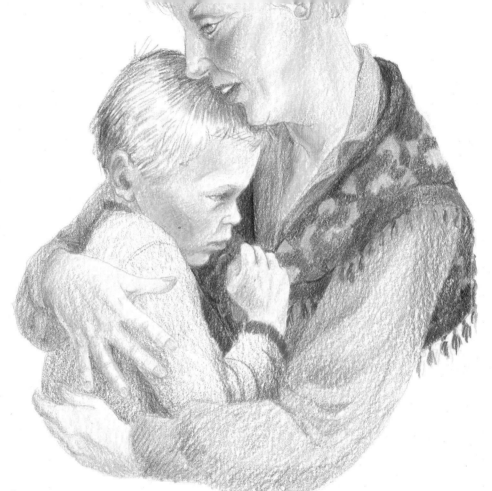

"Do what you can, David. You need to rest more than most kids, but don't give up fighting this disease."

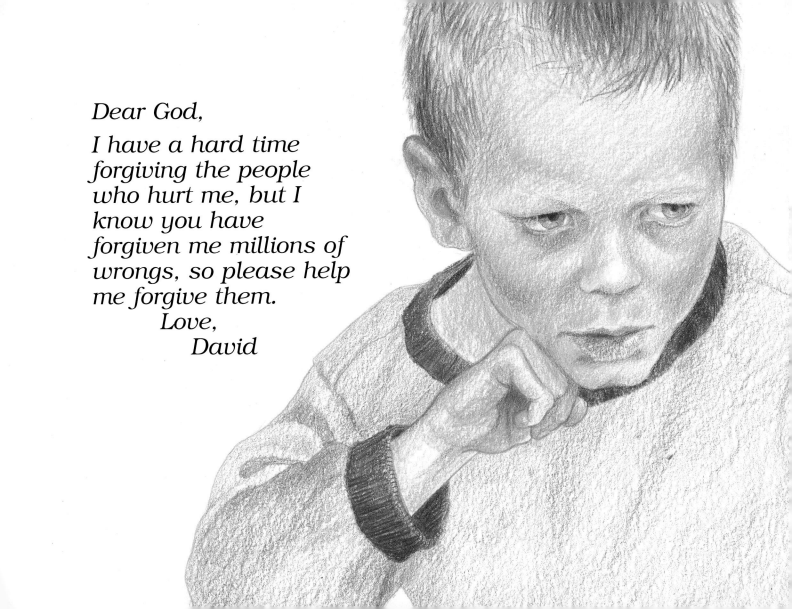

Dear God,

I have a hard time forgiving the people who hurt me, but I know you have forgiven me millions of wrongs, so please help me forgive them.
Love,
David

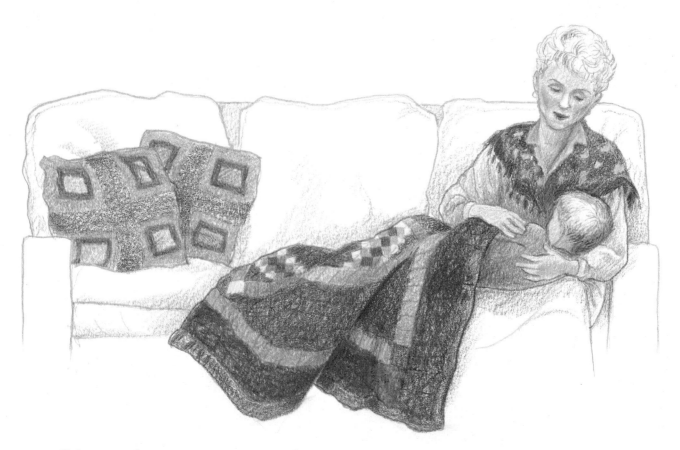

"Grandma, my mouth is sore, my head hurts, my tummy hurts. I'm so tired of being sick."

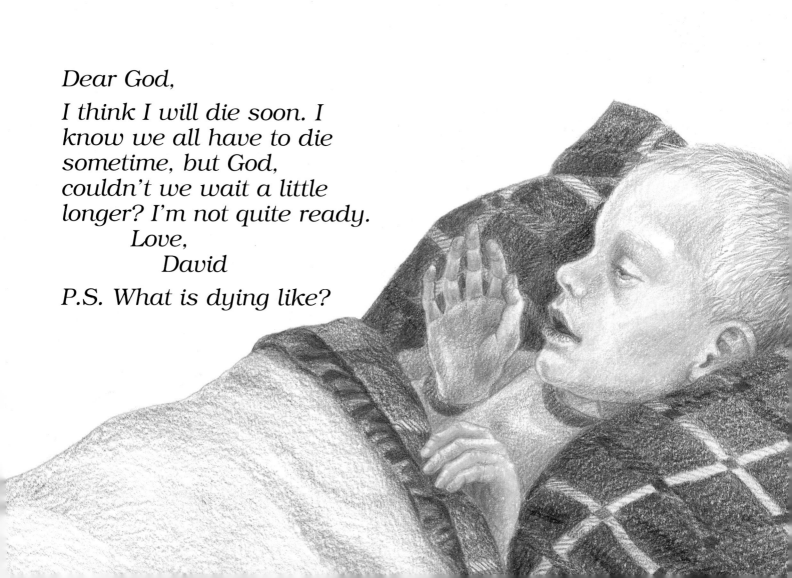

Dear God,

I think I will die soon. I
know we all have to die
sometime, but God,
couldn't we wait a little
longer? I'm not quite ready.
            Love,
                David

P.S. What is dying like?

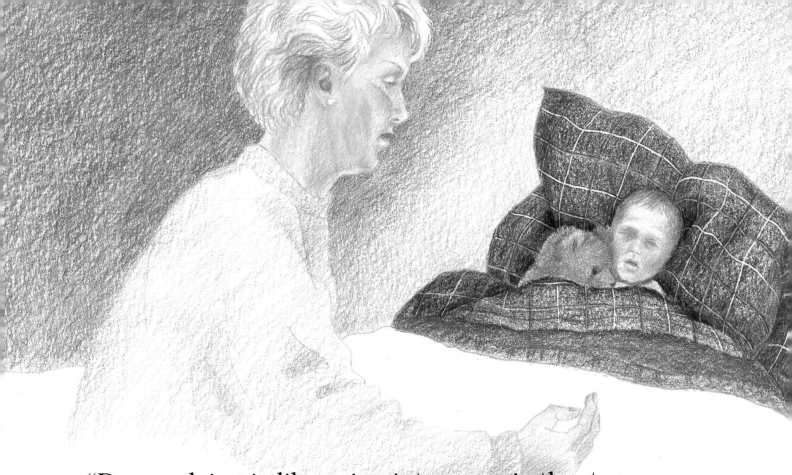

"Davey, dying is like going into a movie theater early and seeing the end of the story before you see the rest, and then staying to watch the movie from the beginning."

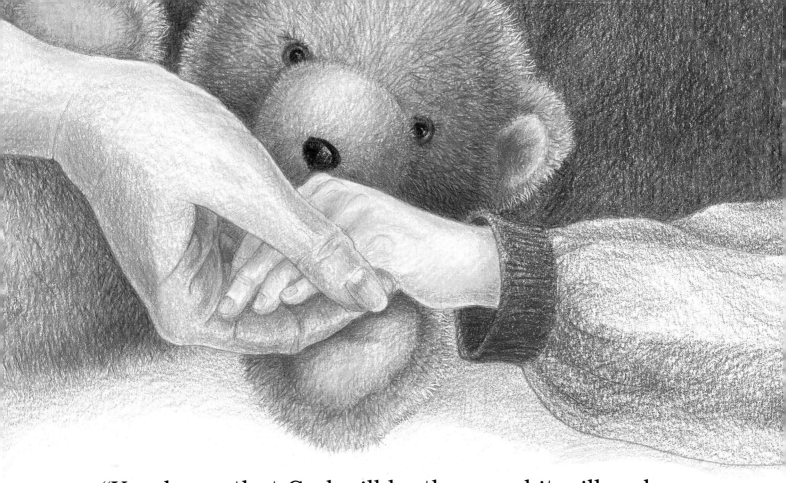

"You know that God will be there and it will end well. You just don't know what will happen *first.*"

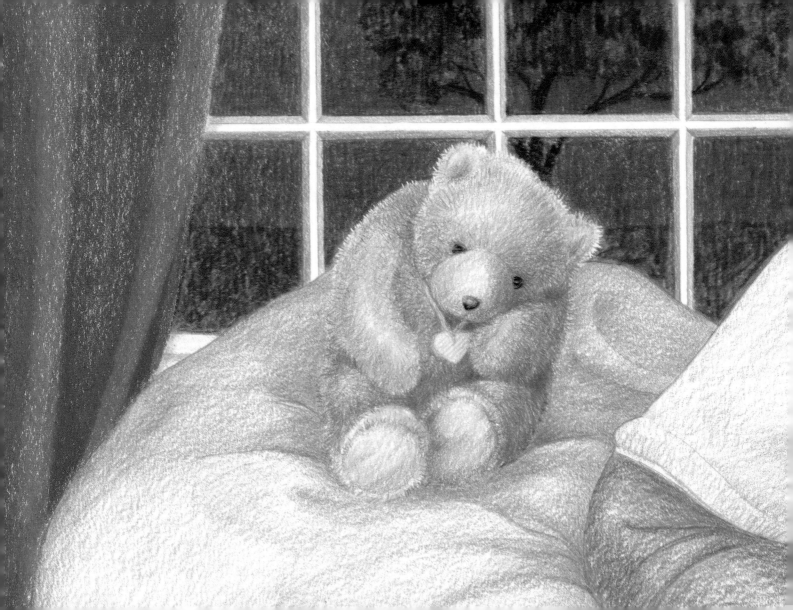

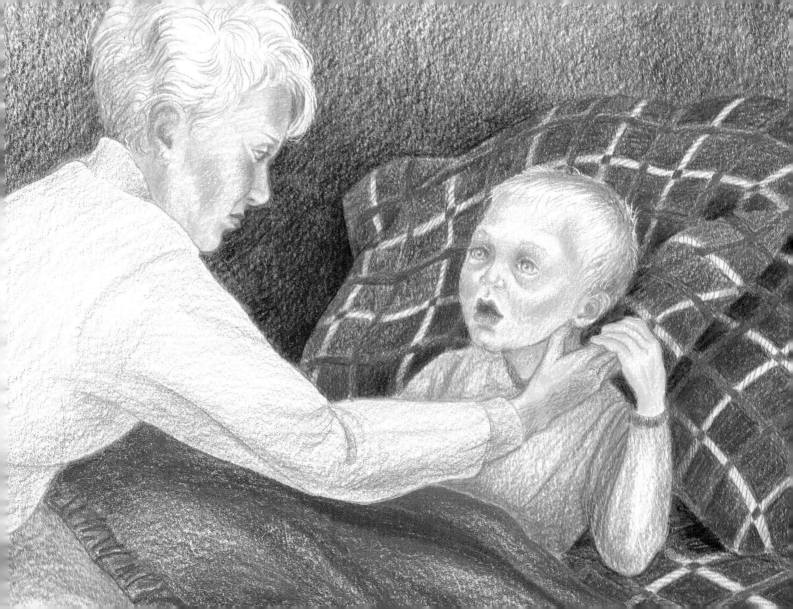

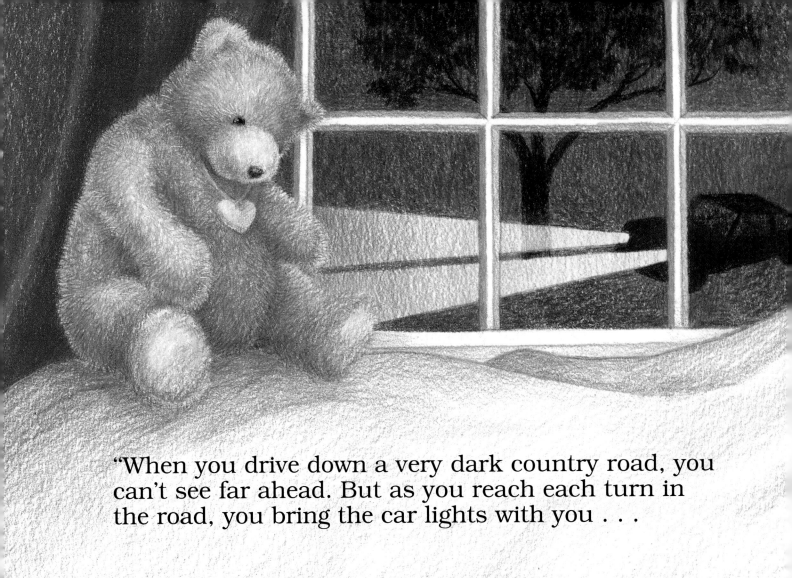

"When you drive down a very dark country road, you can't see far ahead. But as you reach each turn in the road, you bring the car lights with you . . .

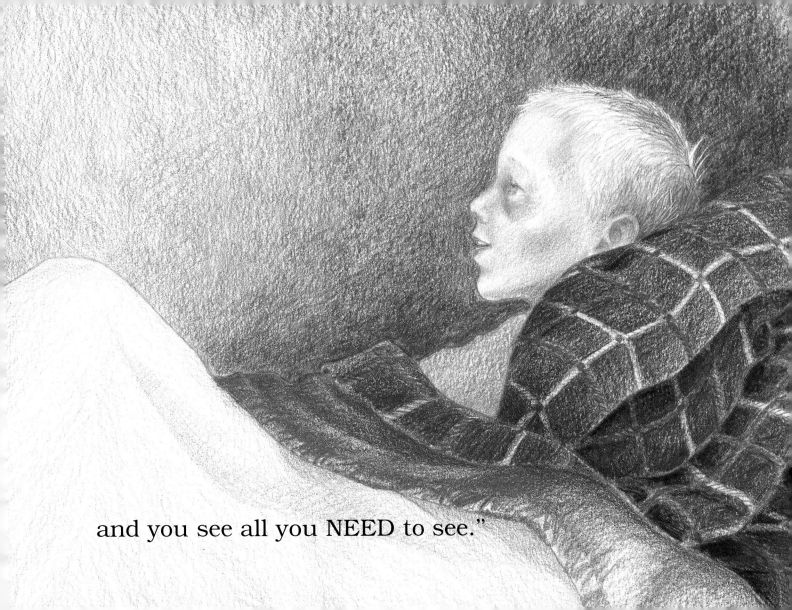

and you see all you NEED to see."

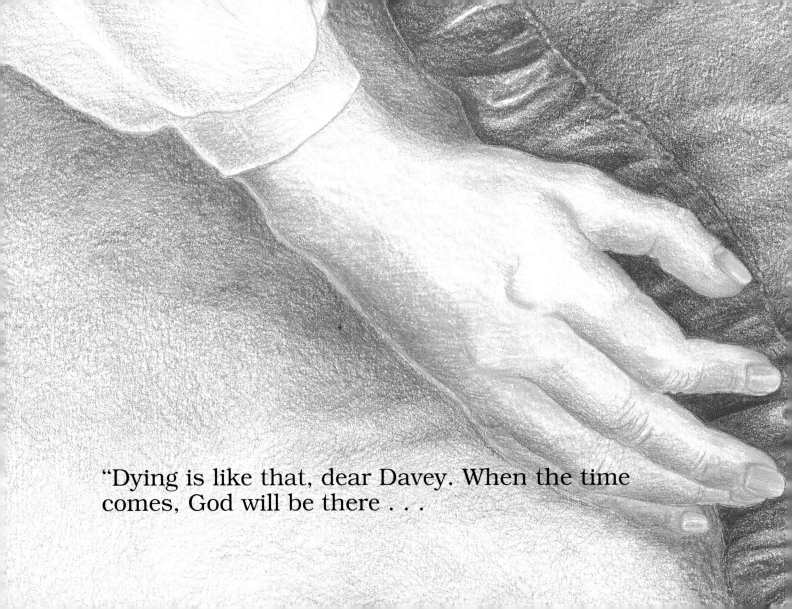

"Dying is like that, dear Davey. When the time comes, God will be there . . .